D1568983

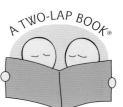
A TWO-LAP BOOK®

Wishing On a Star

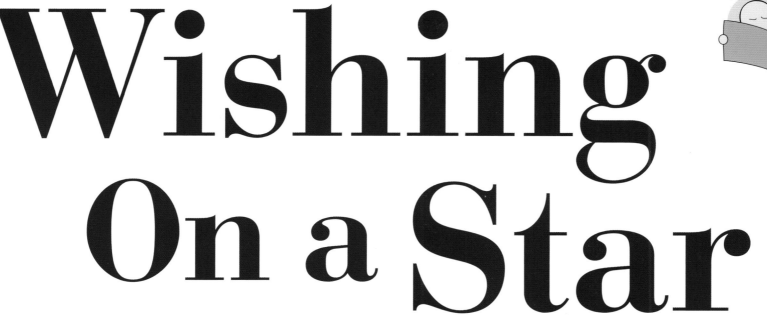

A Read-Aloud Book for Memory-Challenged Adults

by Lydia Burdick
ILLUSTRATED BY JANE FREEMAN

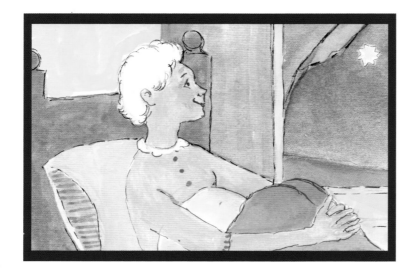

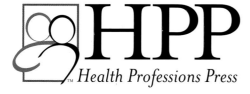
HPP
Health Professions Press

Baltimore • London • Sydney

Additional Two-Lap Books®

The following Two-Lap Books® are also available

The Sunshine on My Face

Happy New Year to You!

To order, contact Health Professions Press, Inc.
Post Office Box 10624
Baltimore, Maryland 21285-0624
410-337-9585
www.healthpropress.com

In loving memory of—

Shirley and Larry Burdick, my parents

Evan Ahern, my brother-in-law

and treasured family and friends—
Dutch Bucher, Sally Breitman, John Pacheco,
Jean Goldin, Chris Senna, Irene Nolt, Gerry Bucher

I dedicate this book to all of you who wish upon a star for the well-being
of your loved ones, and who love them just the way they are.

—Lydia Burdick

For my sisters—Lindy, Lizzy, and Katie—with love!

—Jane Freeman

From the Author

There is something intimate and magical about reading a book together. You can savor this pleasure when you read *Wishing On a Star* with a loved one who has memory loss.

Two-Lap Books® are designed for intimacy; the books are large enough to be spread across two laps. They are written and illustrated to relate to most people's lives—present and past.

I wrote the first book in this series, *The Sunshine on My Face*, for my mother, Shirley Burdick, who was diagnosed with Alzheimer's disease. I wanted to give her words to say and pictures to look at that related to her life as it was at the time. I also wanted to give us a happy activity to do together. My goal was to see a smile on her face with every page.

When I sat down that first time with my mother and with the materials that would become *The Sunshine on My Face*, I didn't know if she would read these sentences to herself, out loud to me, or at all. My mother had been answering our questions only in monosyllables for some time and did not initiate any conversation on her own.

To my delight, with gentle prompting and encouragement, my mother read all the words I presented to her, out loud. There was recognition and pleasure in her voice and bigger smiles than I had seen in years. My written words and the illustrations served as a bridge between us. I had achieved my goal.

I have been thrilled to hear from so many family and professional caregivers about the joyful experiences they have had reading *The Sunshine on My Face* and *Happy New Year to You!* with loved ones, patients, and clients who have memory loss. I hope that *Wishing On a Star*, the latest book in the Two-Lap Books® series, will provide you and your reading partner with similar wonderful rewards.

—Lydia Burdick

How to Use This Book

GETTING STARTED

Tell your reading partner that you have a book you think he or she will enjoy. Get comfortable together. Sit close enough for the book to cover both of your laps. If this is not possible, position yourselves so the book is easily accessible for both of you.

READING TOGETHER

If you think your companion is able to read, invite him or her to read the words to you. You might say, "Mom, I'd love you to read this page to me" or "Mr. Smith, I'll read this page and you read the next, okay?" If you don't get a positive response, be patient. Ask the person to read a few times, always with a smile and without any pressure. It might take awhile for the other person to get involved in the activity—be encouraging.

You can read the words out loud together. If your partner does not wish to read or is not able to read, then read the book out loud to him or her.

You can read this book together from cover to cover several times, read it through once, read a few favorite pages, or read just one page—whatever you and your reading companion choose to do.

Talk with your partner about the sentences. For any page you can ask the person if he/she likes what is described. Ask simple questions about the pictures and the themes. How do they relate to life today or in the past? If you need more suggestions, you will find conversation prompts at the end of the book.

You can also read the book as a group activity, taking turns reading the content and asking questions about it.

LOOKING AT THE ILLUSTRATIONS

Take time to enjoy the pictures and talk about what you see. Sometimes you may want to talk about the pictures alone, without reading the text.

SINGING TOGETHER

Singing is a wonderful activity that triggers happy memories and brings people together. Many songs are brought to mind by the pictures, actions, and characters on each page. Some suggested songs for each page are provided with the conversation prompts at the end of the book. Sing the songs you enjoy and bring music into this activity.

PLAYING GAMES

Many characters and objects repeat in the pictures. Play the game "find the dog," for example, in each scene.

READING LONG-DISTANCE

You and your reading partner can read a Two-Lap Book® out loud over the phone to a family member or friend. It can be a thrill from long distance to hear the voice of a loved one when he or she has mostly stopped talking.

ENJOYING YOUR TIME TOGETHER

Let this book be the spark for an enjoyable and meaningful time together.

Happy reading!

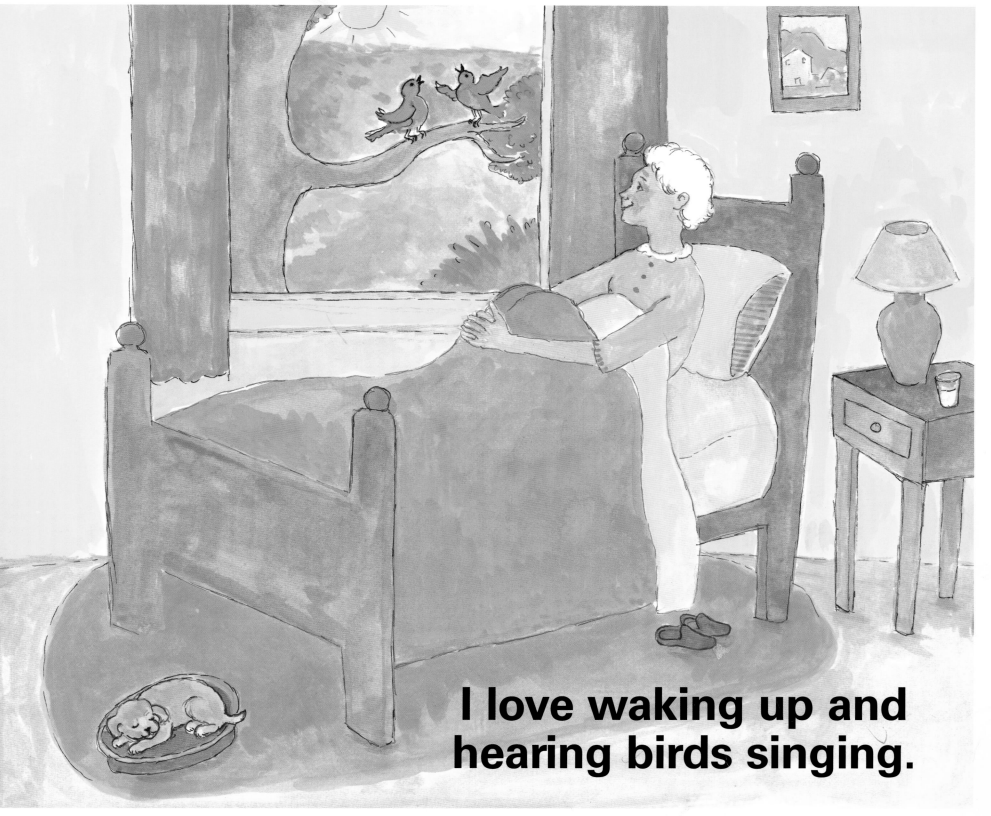

I love waking up and hearing birds singing.

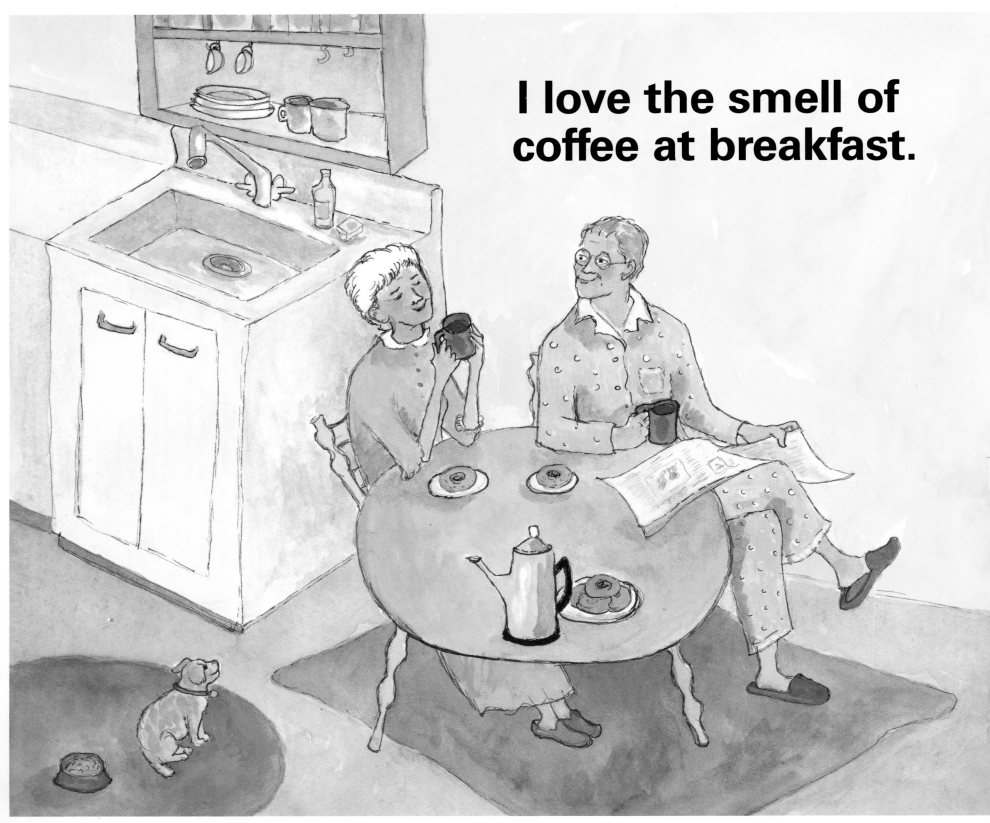

I love the smell of coffee at breakfast.

I love laughing out loud.

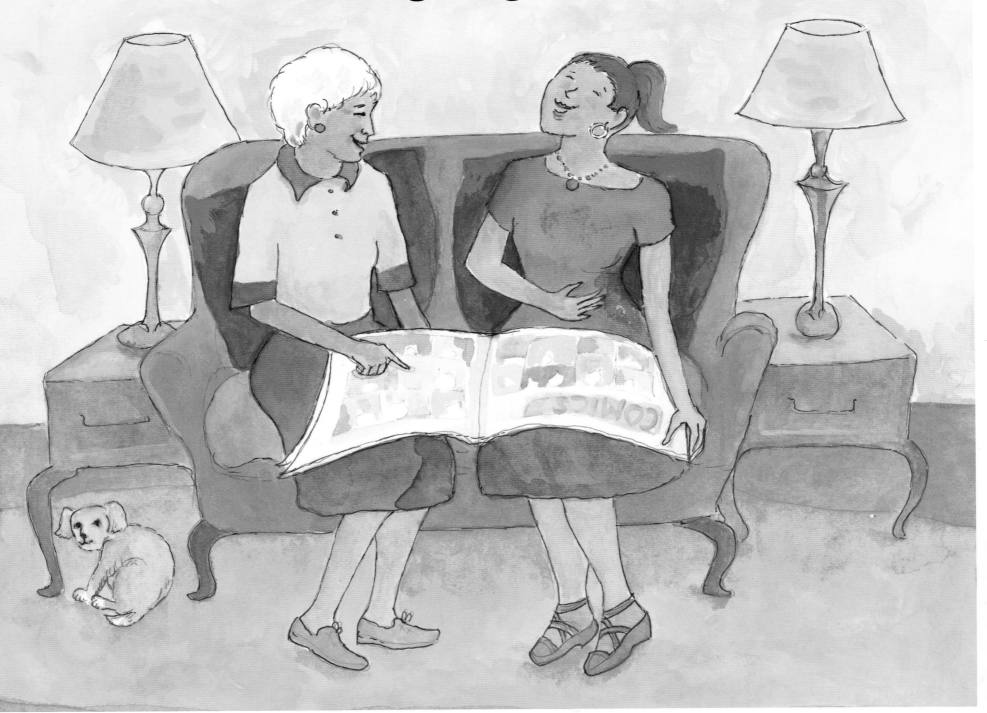

I love telling stories
about the good old days.

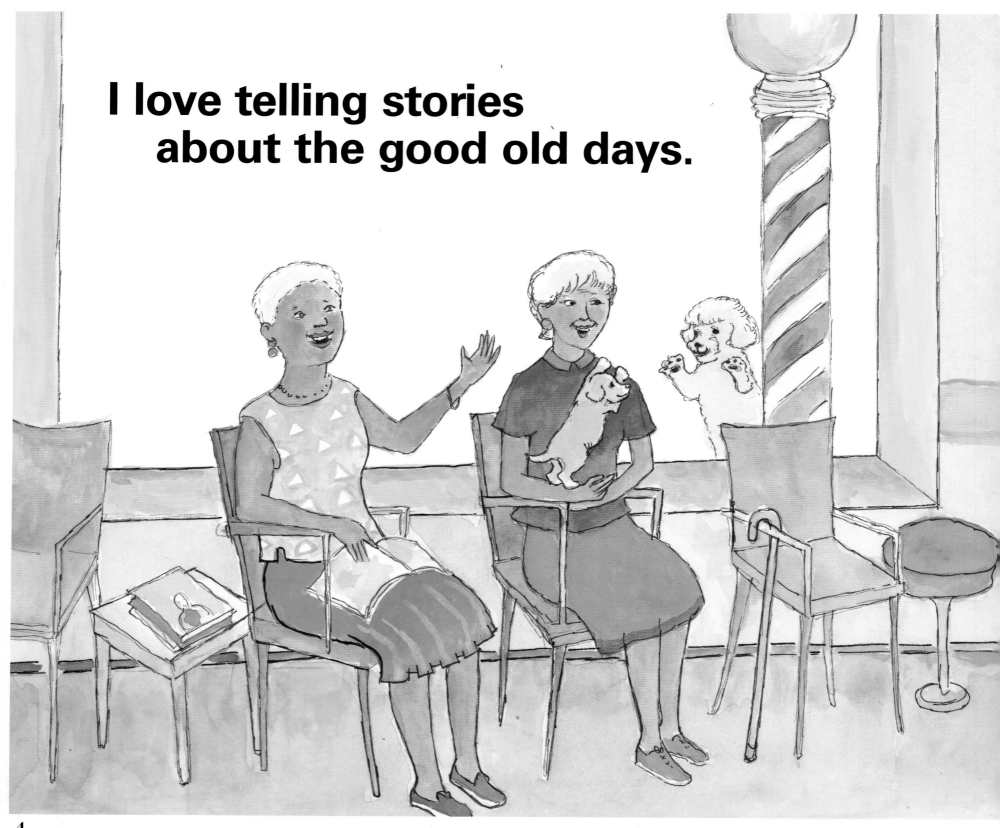

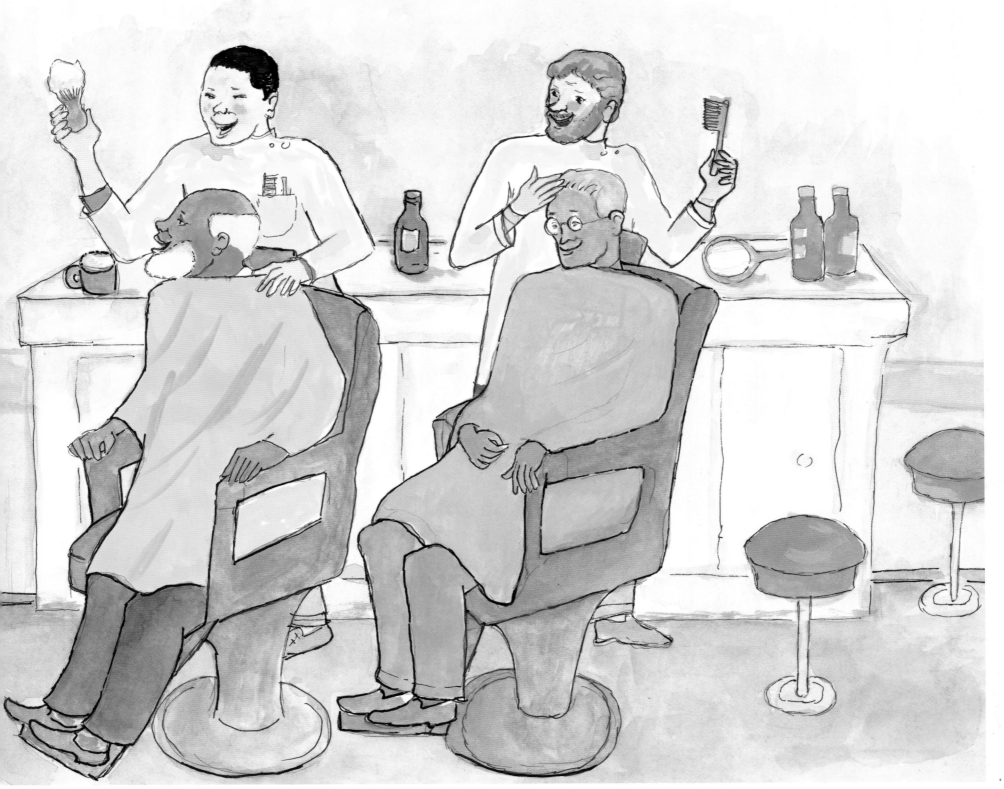

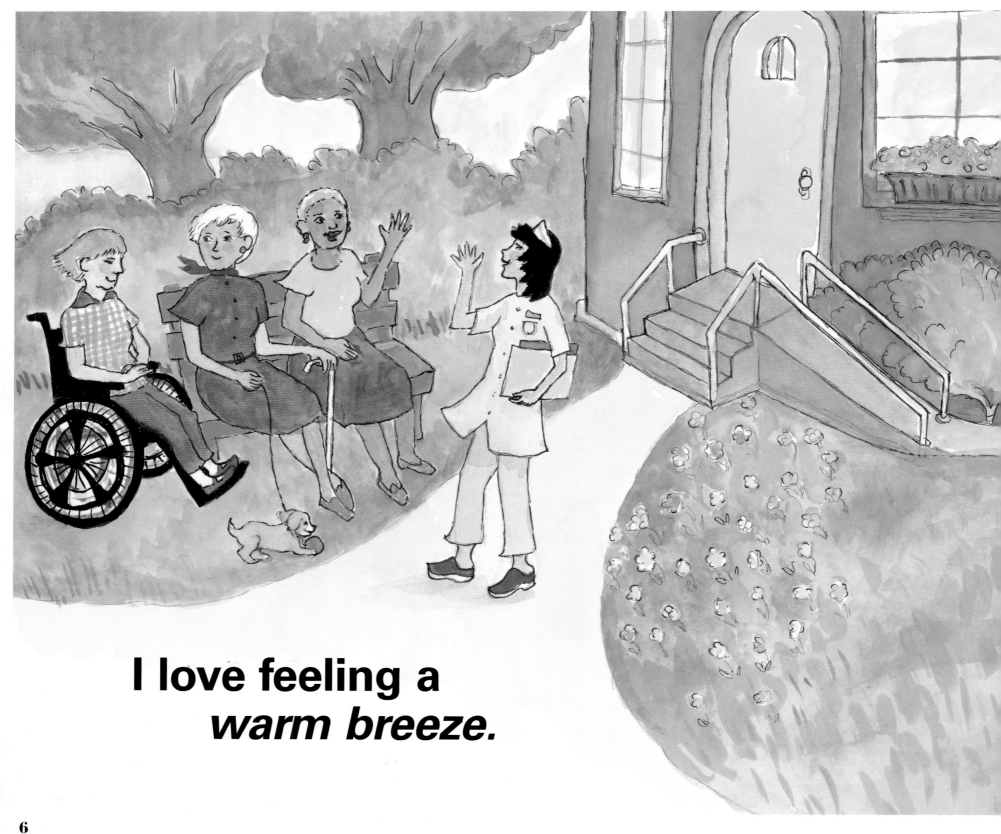

I love feeling a *warm breeze.*

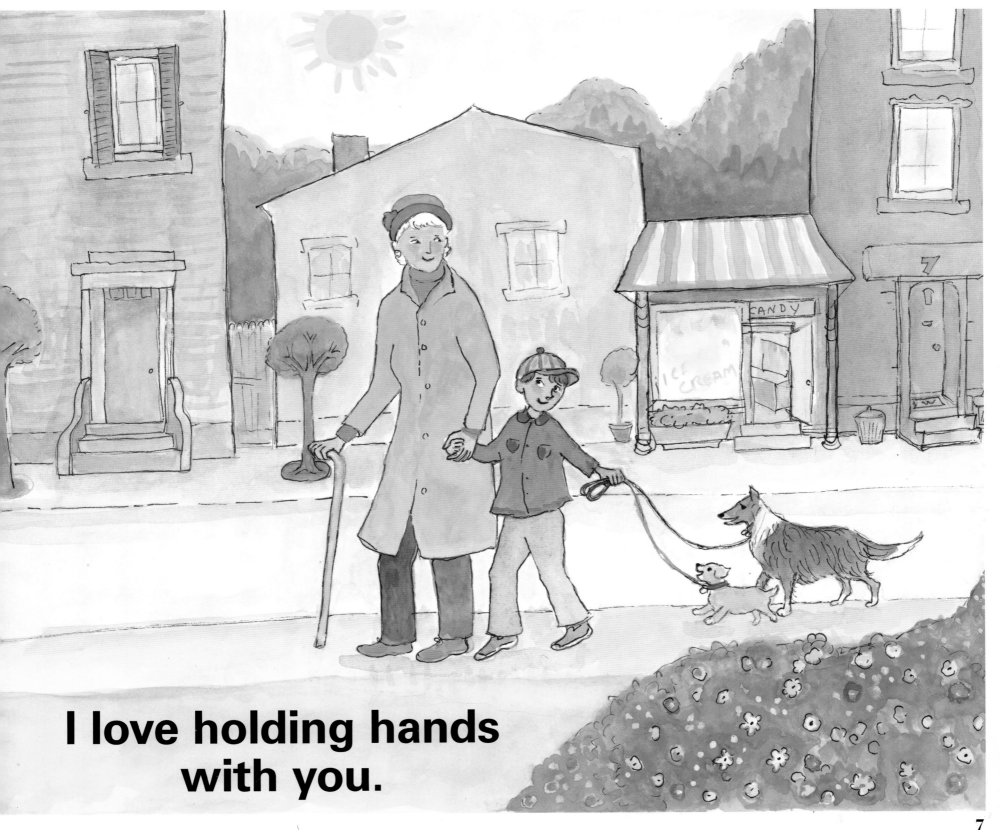

I love holding hands
with you.

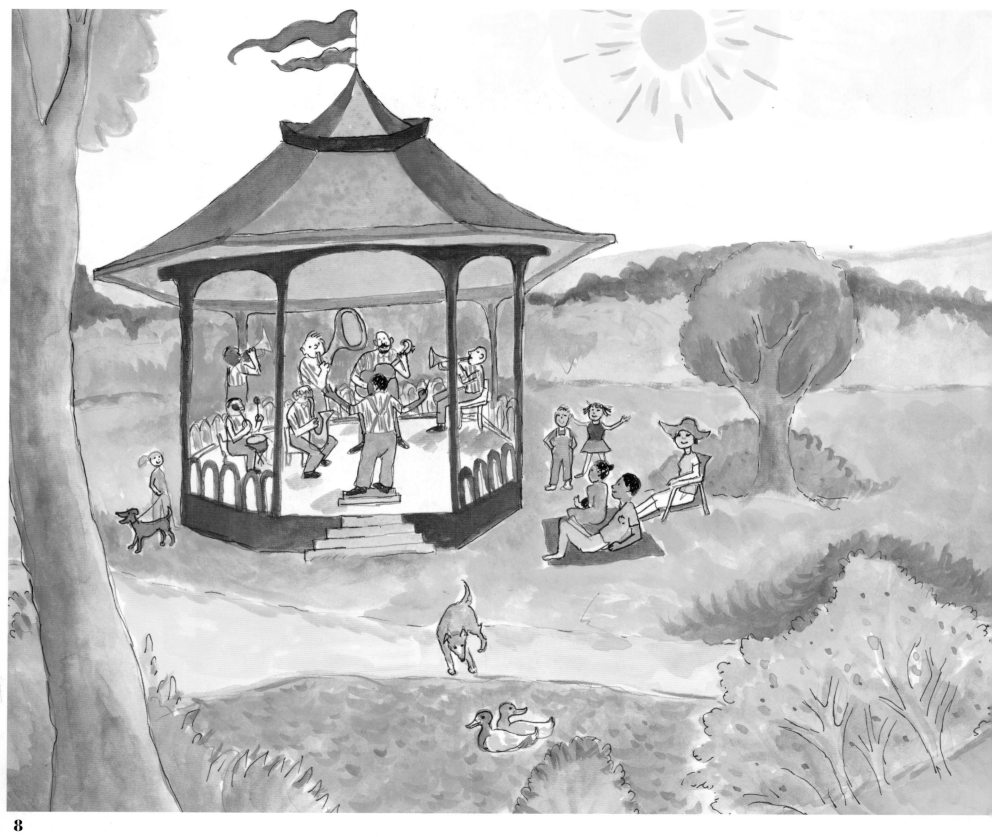

I love hearing wonderful music.

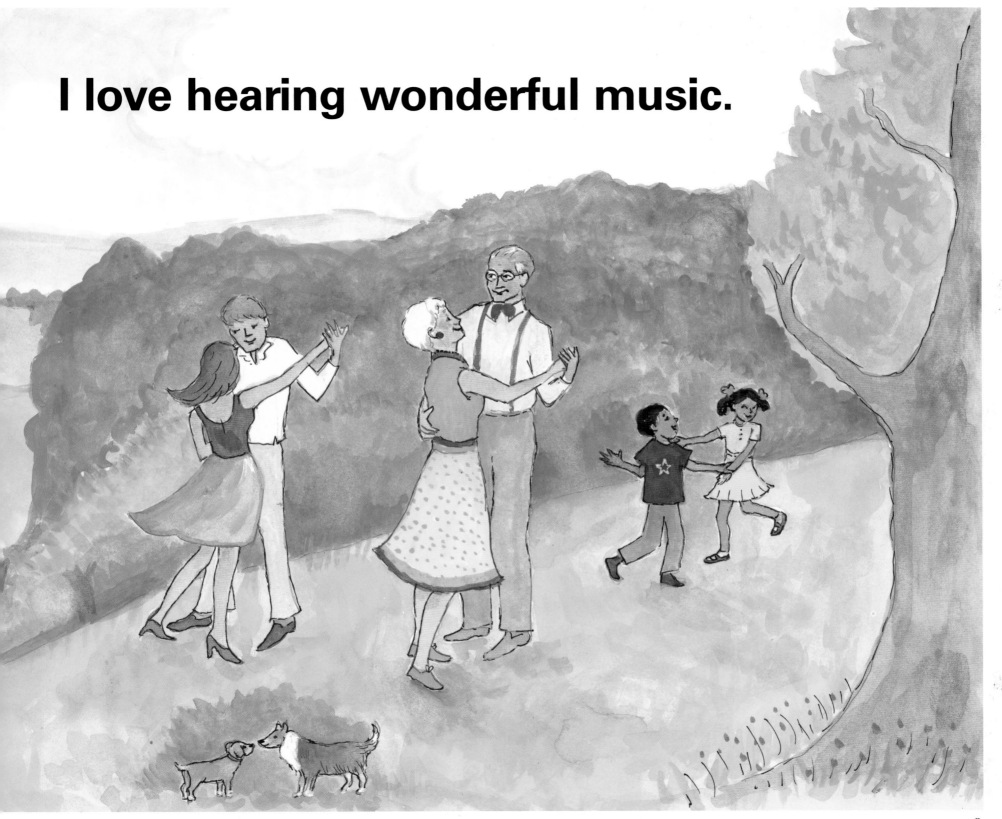

I love visiting
with my family.

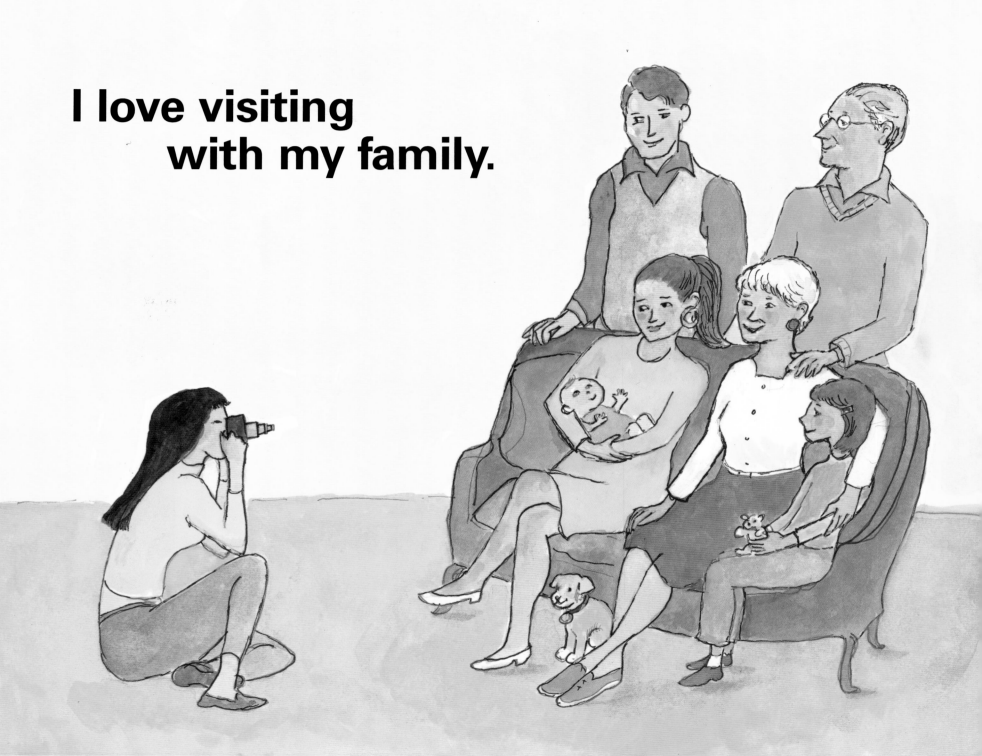

I love putting pictures in my photo album.

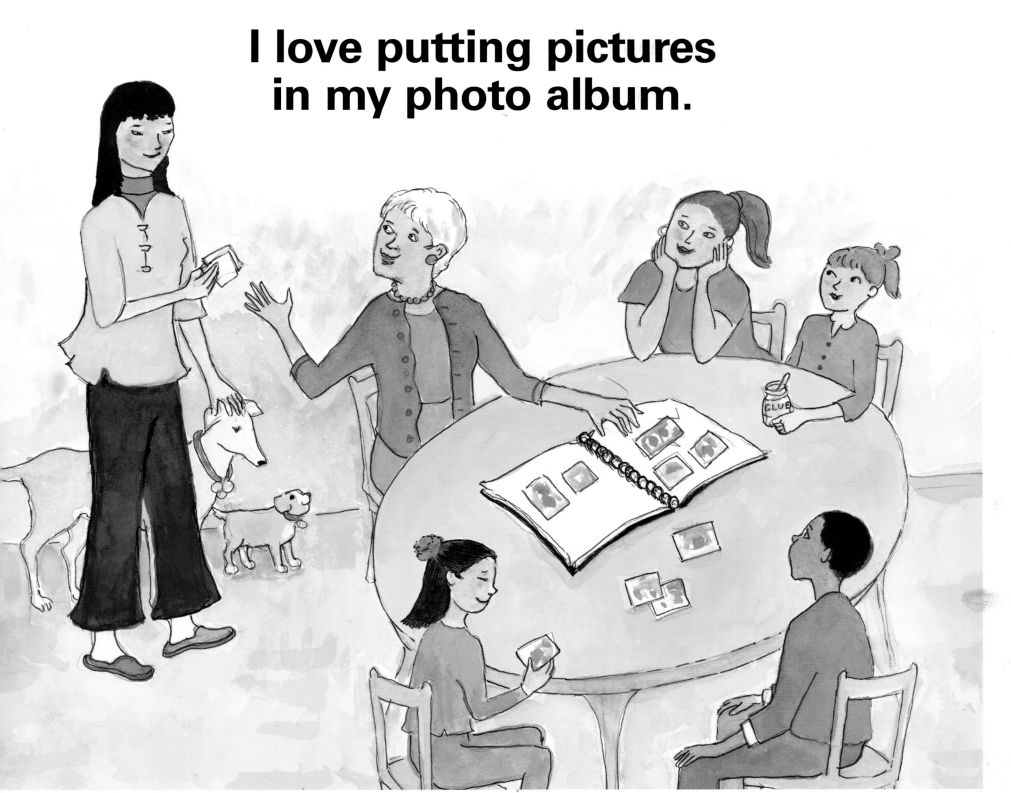

I love finding a rainbow in the sky.

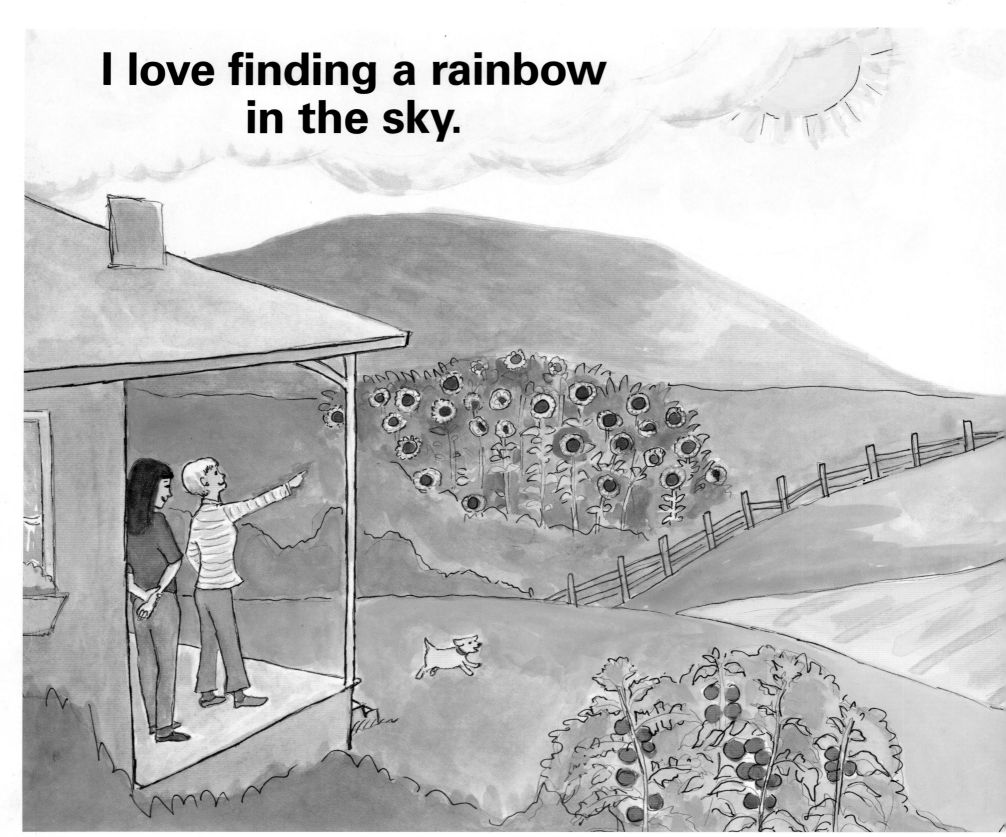

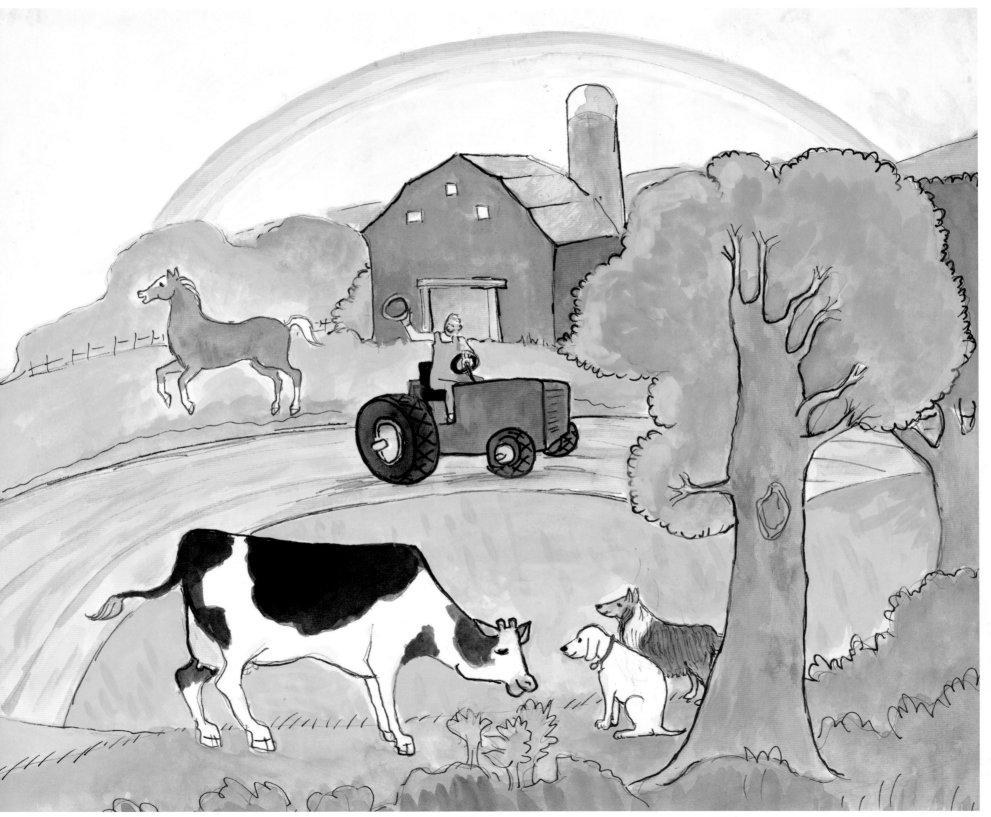

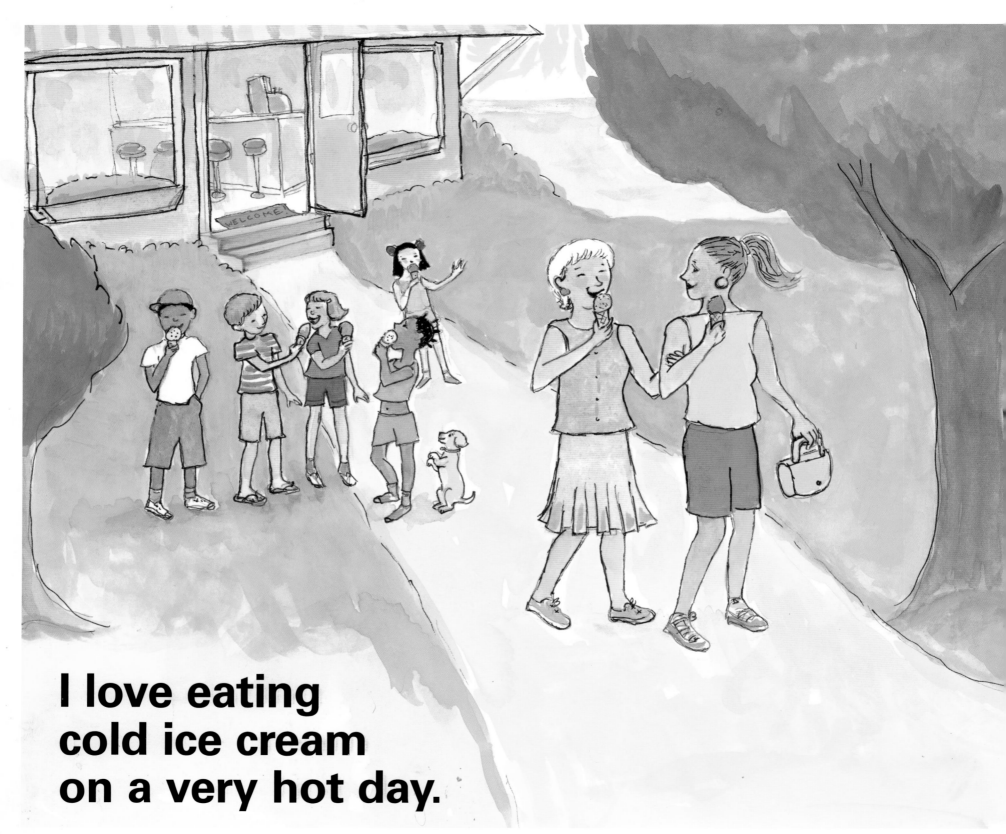

I love eating
cold ice cream
on a very hot day.

I love playing with my pet.

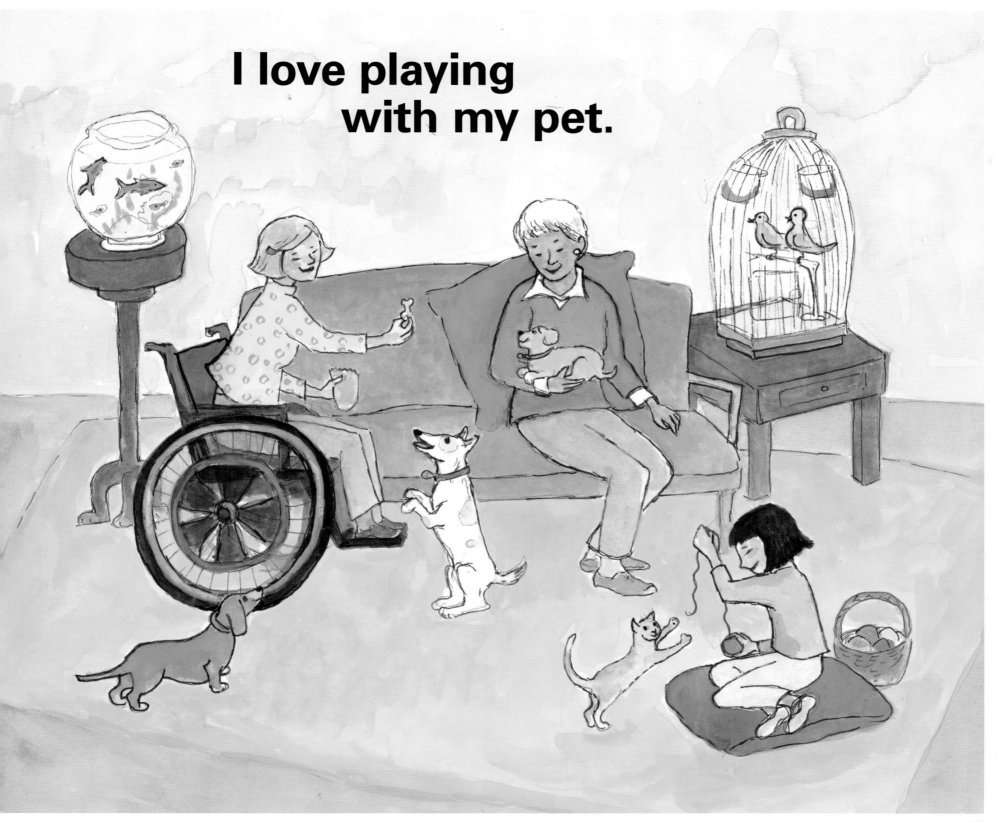

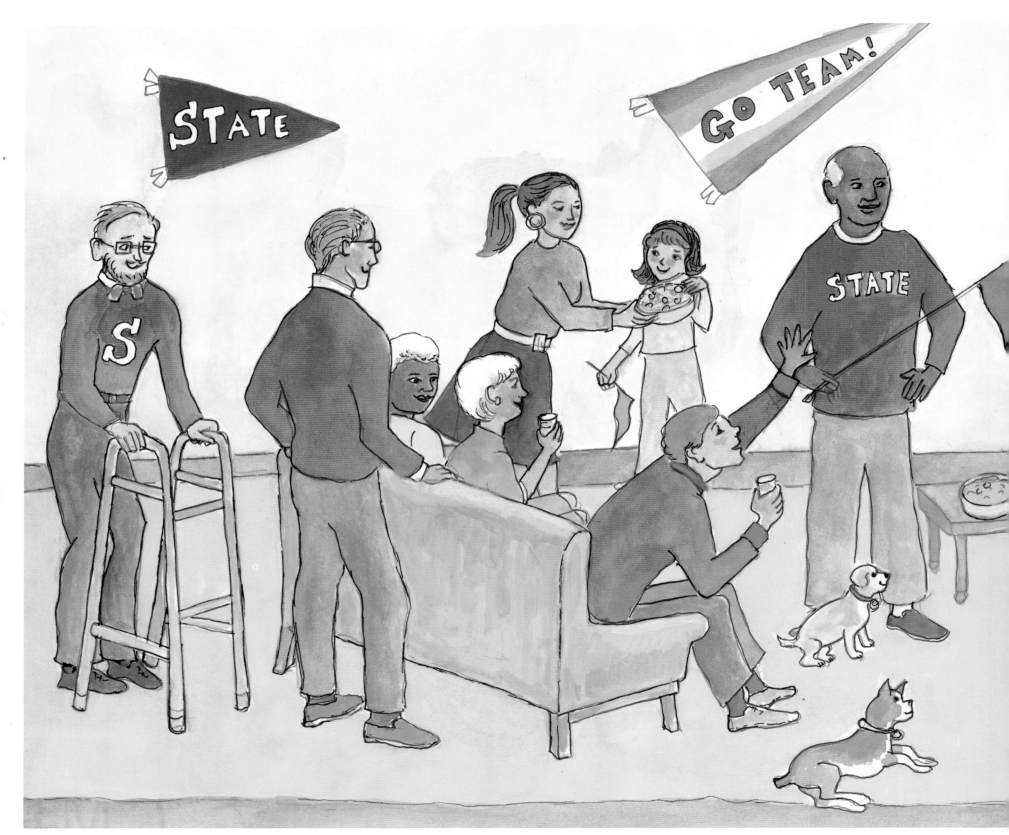

I love cheering for my favorite team!

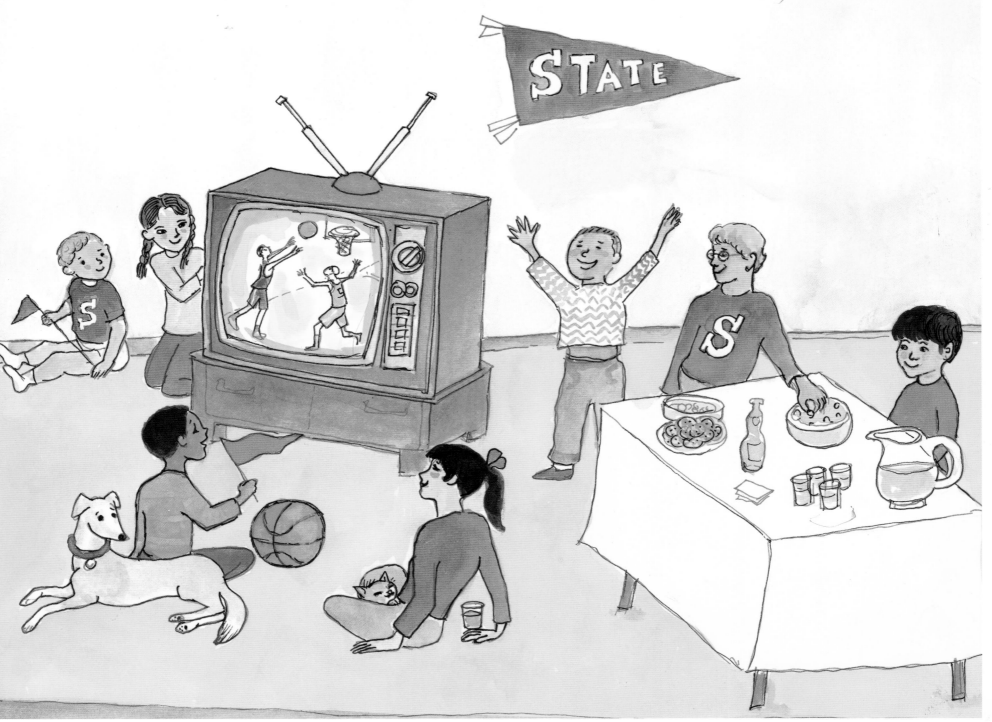

I love seeing you smile.

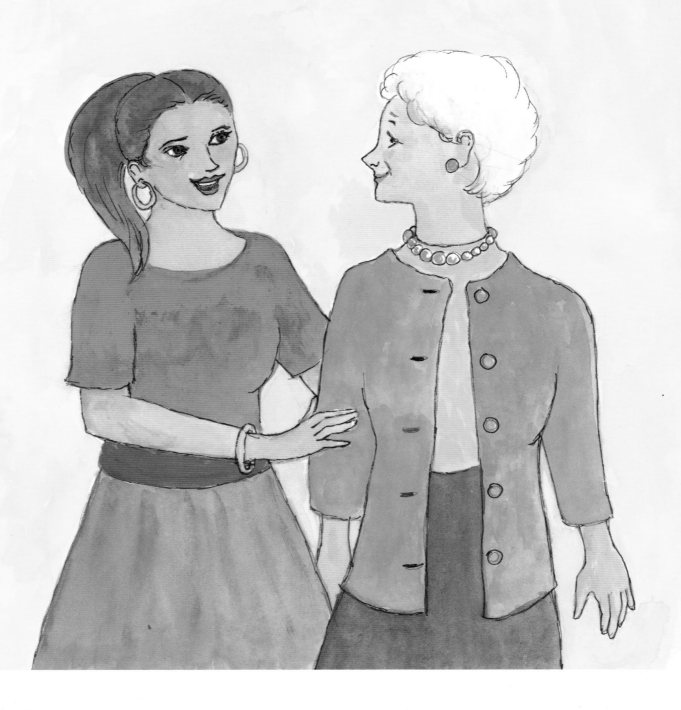

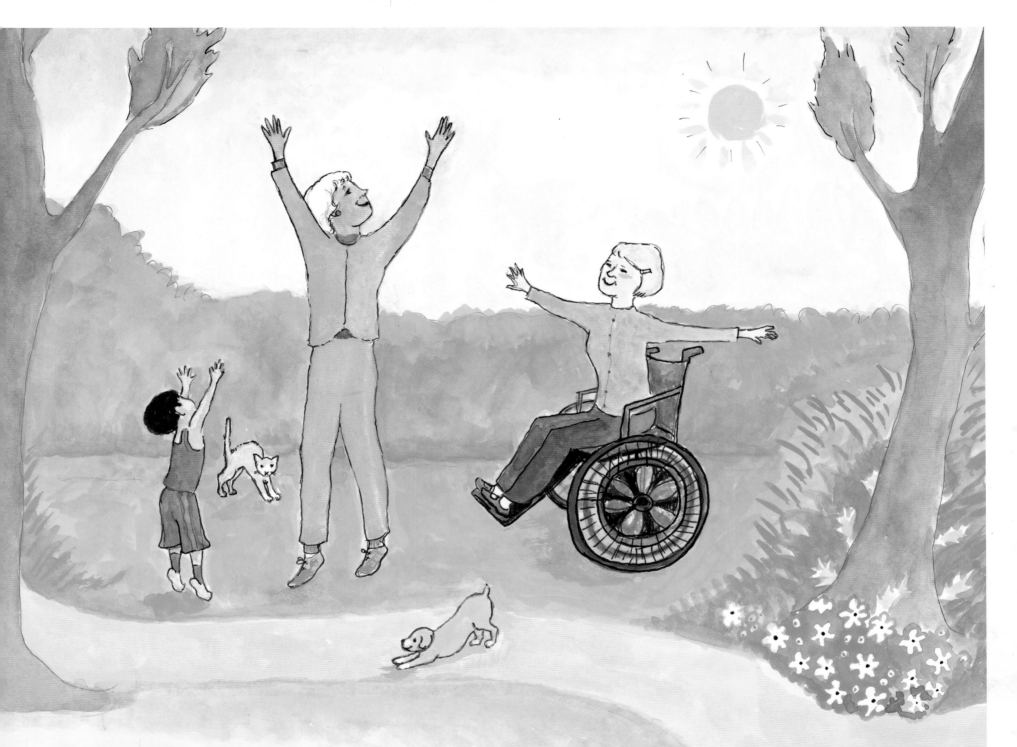

I love having a good stretch.

I love singing
my favorite songs.

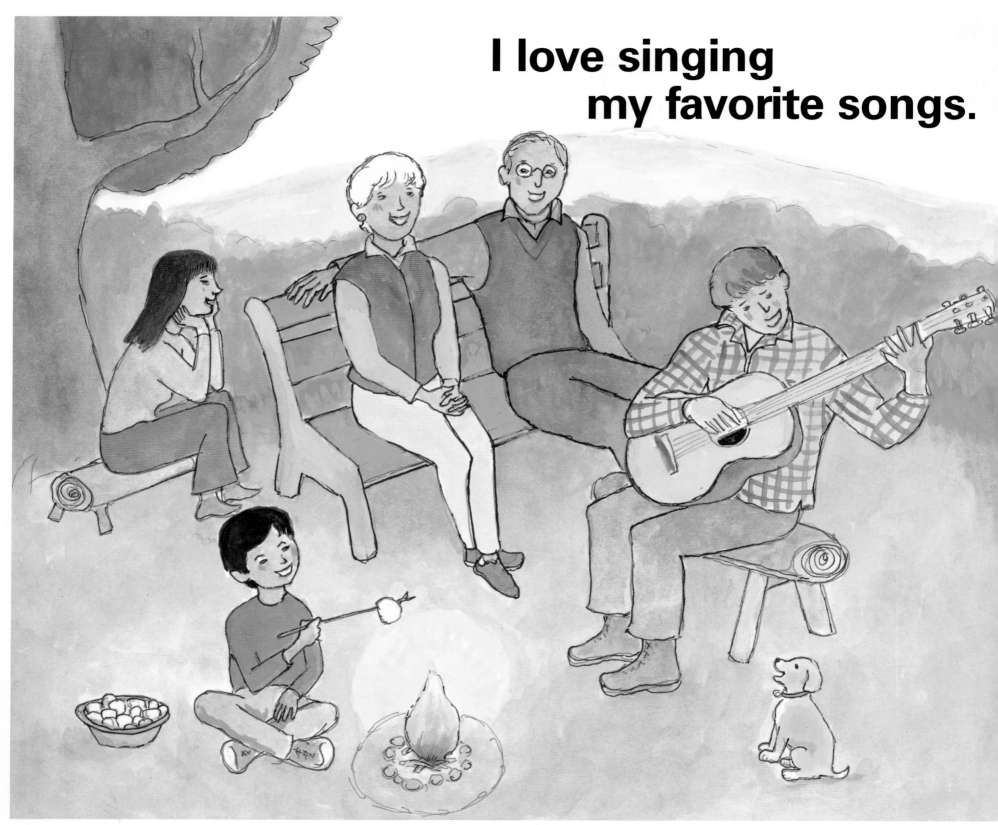

I love giving thanks
at the end of the day.

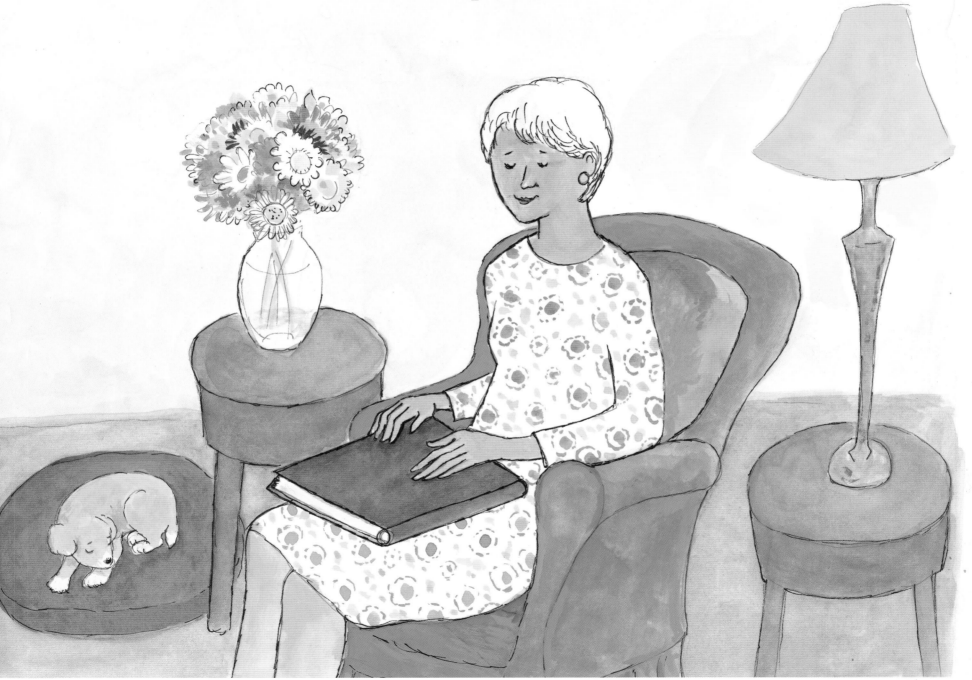

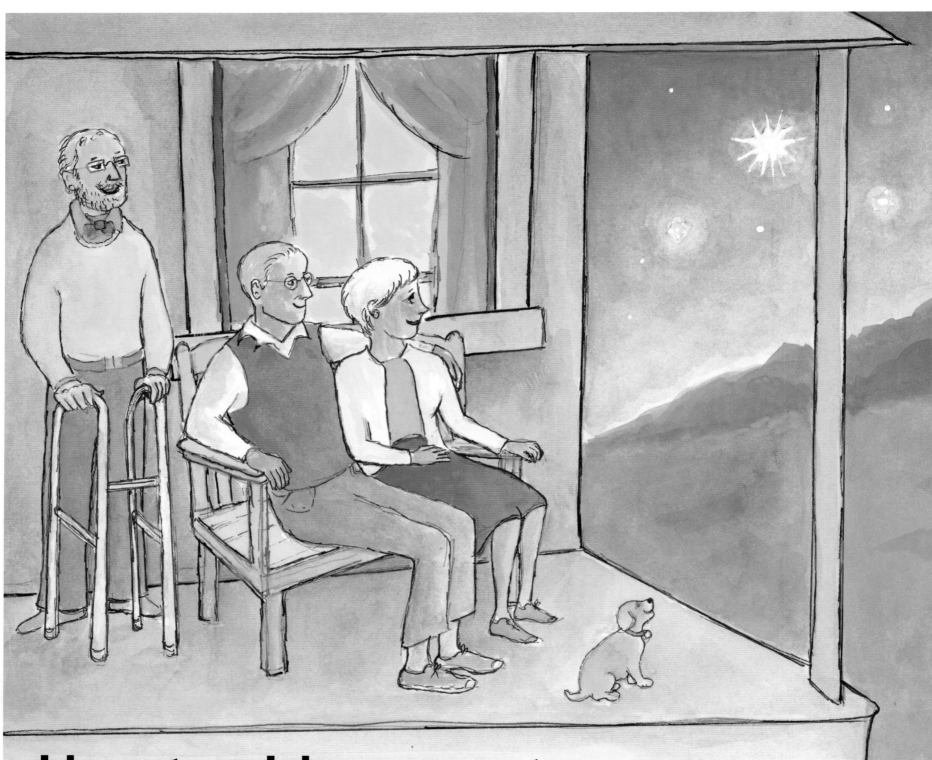

I love to wish upon a star.

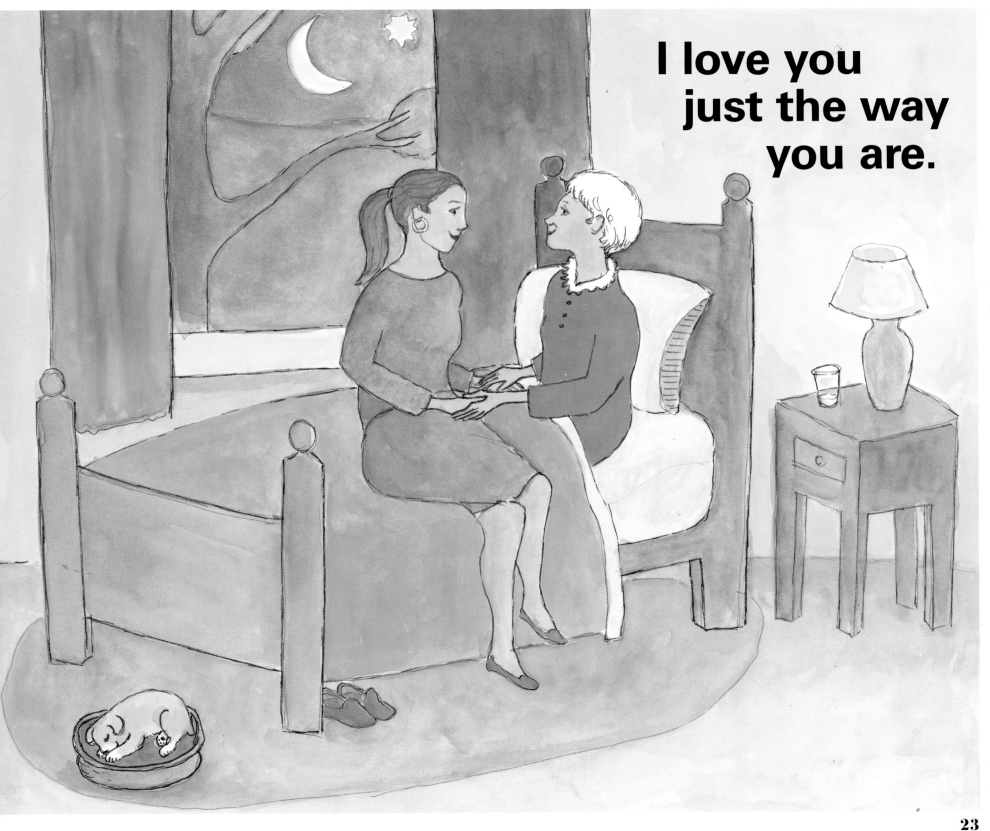

I love you
just the way
you are.

23

Sample Conversation Prompts and Songs for Each Page

Page 1   **I love waking up and hearing birds singing.**

How do you feel when you wake up?
Do you like to hear birds singing?
Do you like to wake up early or late?

Songs: *Oh, What a Beautiful Morning!*
    When the Red, Red Robin Comes Bob, Bob, Bobbin' Along
    Oh! How I Hate to Get Up in the Morning!

Pages 2   **I love the smell of coffee at breakfast.**

Are you a coffee drinker? A tea drinker?
Do you drink your coffee black or with cream and sugar?
What do you like to eat for breakfast?

Songs: *I Love Coffee, I Love Tea*
    Tea for Two
    Sugartime

Pages 3   **I love laughing out loud.**

Do you like to laugh?
What makes you laugh?
Are you ticklish?

Song: *I Love to Laugh*

Pages 4–5   **I love telling stories about the good old days.**

Where did you grow up?
Tell me about something that you did in your life.
What was the best time of your life?

Songs: *Those Were the Days, My Friend*
    Try to Remember

Page 6   **I love feeling a warm breeze.**

How does a warm breeze make you feel?
What does a warm breeze make you think of?
How does a cold wind make you feel?

Songs: *Summertime*
    Those Lazy, Hazy, Crazy Days of Summer
    Autumn Breeze

Page 7   **I love holding hands with you.**

Would you like to hold my hand?
Who do you like to hold hands with?
How do you feel when you hold hands?

Songs: *I Want to Hold Your Hand*
    Walking My Baby Back Home
    Stranger in Paradise

Page 8–9   **I love hearing wonderful music.**

What kind of music do you like?
Would you like to listen to some music now?
Do you/did you play a musical instrument?

Songs: *The Sound of Music*
    As Long as I'm Singing
    Put Another Nickel In

Page 10   **I love visiting with my family.**

Who is in your family?
Do you like visiting with your family?
Who else do you like to visit with?

Songs: *Swanee*
    Over the River and Through the Woods
    There's No Place Like Home for the Holidays
    Home, Home On the Range

Pages 11   **I love putting pictures in my photo album.**

Do you like to take pictures?
Do you have a photo album?
Would you like to look at your photo album?

Songs: *Memories Are Made of This*
    Memories of You
    As Time Goes By

Pages 12–13   I love finding a rainbow in the sky.

How do you feel when you see a rainbow?
Do you believe there is a pot of gold at the end of a rainbow?
Do you like it when it's raining outside? Do you like it when it's sunny?

Songs: *Somewhere Over the Rainbow*
         Look for the Silver Lining
         Come Rain or Come Shine

Pages 14   I love eating cold ice cream on a very hot day.

Do you like to eat ice cream?
What flavor do you like?
Do you like it when it's very hot outside?

Song: *Summertime*

Cheer: I scream, you scream, we all scream for ice cream!

Page 15   I love playing with my pet.

Do you/did you have pets?
Did you live around animals?
What kinds of animals do you like?

Songs: *How Much Is That Doggie in the Window?*
         Old McDonald Had a Farm

Page 16–17   I love cheering for my favorite team!

Do you have a favorite sports team?
Do you like to watch sports on TV? Which sport?
Did you play a sport when you were growing up?

Songs: *Take Me Out to the Ballgame*
         Hail, Hail the Gang's All Here
         Specific school songs

Page 18   I love seeing you smile.

Doesn't it feel good to smile?
Can you give me a big smile?
Do you know I love to see you smile?

Songs: *When You're Smiling*
         If You're Happy and You Know It
         Pack Up Your Troubles in Your Old Kit Bag

Page 19   I love having a good stretch.

Does it feel good to stretch?
Do you like to stretch when you wake up?
Can we try a stretch now?

Song: *Head, Shoulders, Knees, and Toes*

Page 20   I love singing my favorite songs.

Would you like to sing one of your favorite songs now?
Have you ever sat around a campfire singing songs?
Do you like roasting marshmallows? S'mores?

Songs: *Kumbaya*
         We'll Sing in the Sunshine
         Singing in the Rain

Page 21   I love giving thanks at the end of the day.

What are your thankful for?
Who are you thankful for?
Let's talk about who is thankful for you.

Songs: *We Gather Together*
         I Believe

Page 22   I love to wish upon a star.

Have you ever wished on a star? What do you wish for?
What do you think about when you look at the stars?

Songs: *When You Wish Upon a Star*
         Twinkle, Twinkle, Little Star
         Catch a Falling Star

Poem: *Starlight, star bright, first star I see tonight . . .*

Page 23   I love you just the way you are.

Do you like to hear me say "I love you just the way you are"?
How does it feel when someone says they love you?
Who do you want to tell that you love them?

Songs: *A Bushel and a Peck*
         Till There Was You
         Goodnight, Sweetheart
         Brahm's Lullaby

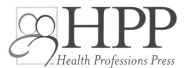

Health Professions Press, Inc.
Post Office Box 10624
Baltimore, MD 21285-0624

www.healthpropress.com

Text copyright © 2009 Lydia Burdick.
Illustrations copyright © 2009 Health Professions Press.
All rights reserved.

A Two-Lap Book® is a trademark owned by Lydia Burdick.

Illustrated by Jane Freeman.

The following Two-Lap Books® are also available from Health Professions Press, Inc.:
The Sunshine on My Face: A Read-Aloud Book for Memory-Challenged Adults
Happy New Year to You! A Read-Aloud Book for Memory Challenged Adults
To order, contact Health Professions Press, Inc. (410-337-9585 or www.healthpropress.com)

Two-Lap Books® are available at a quantity discount with bulk purchases for educational, therapeutic, and human services programs. For information, please write to: SPECIAL SALES DEPARTMENT, HEALTH PROFESSIONS PRESS, POST OFFICE BOX 10624, BALTIMORE, MD 21285 OR FAX 410-337-8539.

Reinforced library binding. Printed in China.

Library of Congress Cataloging-in-Publication Data
Burdick, Lydia.
  Wishing on a star : a read-aloud book for memory-challenged adults / by Lydia Burdick ; illustrated by Jane Freeman.
      p. cm. — (A two-lap book series)
  ISBN 978-1-932529-43-2 (cloth)
  1. Alzheimer's disease—Popular works. 2. Oral reading. 3. Memory disorders in old age. 4. Large-type books. I. Freeman, Jane. II. Title.
  RC523.2.B875 2009
  616.8'31—dc22
                    2009001026

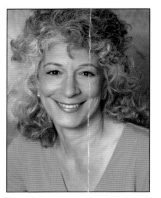

Photograph by Steve Ladner

With a master's degree in Clinical Practices (psychology), Lydia Burdick's career has been in human resources. She has been a consultant in an international outplacement firm since 1993. Lydia conceived the idea for her first Two-Lap Book®, *The Sunshine on My Face: A Read-Aloud Book for Memory-Challenged Adults*, in the course of caring for her mother who was diagnosed with Alzheimer's disease. "One of my greatest pleasures," she says, "was sitting next to my mother and hearing her read the words from this book when she had otherwise stopped speaking almost completely."